What People Are Saying About *Can I Still Kiss You?*

"A sensitive and useful book for all those living with what the author has experienced. It will help you find the courage and strength with which to share your wounds and love."

—Bernie Siegel, M.D.
author, *Love, Medicine & Miracles* and *Prescriptions for Living*

"I often have the opportunity to care for patients with young children, who have found it extremely difficult and awkward to broach the topic of their disease with their kids. This book does an excellent job in reviewing those areas that are the most commonly brought out as concerns by the children. I respect the author's sensitivity and thoughtfulness."

—Neil M. Barth, M.D., F.A.C.P.

"Having worked with families for over fifteen years, I believe this book will be a tremendous help to dads and moms who love their kids and who are looking for a way to talk to their children about cancer and cancer treatments. The format of the book—questions kids have and helpful answers parents can offer—reveals children's core concerns and provides a guide for parents to help their children cope with the feelings and changes in the family that often come with a diagnosis of cancer."

—Margaret Reedy, Ph.D.
clinical psychologist

CAN I STILL KISS YOU?

Answering Your Children's Questions About Cancer

NEIL RUSSELL

Health Communications, Inc.
Deerfield Beach, Florida

www.hci-online.com

Library of Congress Cataloging-in-Publication Data

Russell, Neil

    Can I still kiss you? : answering your children's questions about cancer / Neil Russell.

      p.   cm.

    ISBN 1-55874-928-4 (tradepaper)

    1. Cancer—Miscellanea. 2. Children of cancer patients.
3. Russell, Neil—Health. 4. Cancer—Patients—United States—
Biography. I. Title.

RC262.R87 2001
616.99'4—dc21   2001039448

Publisher: Health Communications, Inc.
                3201 S.W. 15th Street
                Deerfield Beach, FL 33442-8190

Cover photo ©Rubberball Productions
Cover and inside book design by Lawna Patterson Oldfield

For Andrew and Trevor,
whose laughter and love made
the fight worth it.

Love, Dad

CONTENTS

ACKNOWLEDGMENTS

Usually, an author begins by thanking his editor and publisher. I will do so in a moment, but I hope the good folks at Health Communications will understand that, in this case, I need to do something else first.

I met many doctors during my two fights with cancer. Each of them was exceptionally professional and kind to a fault. Four, however, deserve special mention:

Gilbert Goodman, M.D., who has been my physician for the past sixteen years, watched over me through it all. He has that rare quality of making you feel as though you are his only patient.

Ronald Solomon, M.D., the fly fisherman with the ready smile, had a penchant for detail that always made me feel both safe and informed. He gave me the gift of life, and I can never thank him enough.

Neil M. Barth, M.D., F.A.C.P., an incredibly busy oncologist who took the time to read my manuscript and offer wonderful words of encouragement.

And Margaret Reedy, Ph.D., the soft-spoken clinical psychologist who helped me get to the heart of some of the tough questions in this book.

I would also like to thank Hilda Knight, Dr. Goodman's nurse and an unfailing, beaming optimist who is always genuinely happy to see everyone; and Sarah LaFlamme, Dr. Solomon's right hand, a cancer survivor herself, who understood and encouraged me through the tough times.

And most of all, I want to thank the professionals of the Hoag Hospital Surgical Unit and the Hoag Cancer Center in Newport Beach, California. Expressing how much I appreciate what they did is impossible.

And in the way I would not have been here

today without the people mentioned above, this book would not be in your hands without Peter Vegso, the president of HCI, who was unfailingly gracious in our dealings. And Christine Belleris and Allison Janse, my editors, who embraced this project and pushed it through the HCI process, then hung in there with an often obtuse and always slow writer. Erica Orloff, my other editor—clearly, I needed a great deal of help—is responsible for helping me set the right tone for the book.

I would also like to thank four people for being a part of my life: my wife, Sandi, whose father succumbed to cancer last year after a long and difficult battle and whose mother is a cancer survivor; my sister, Marsha, who just completed treatment for cancer; my mother, Dorothy, who fought her own battle with the disease; and my father, Ralph, who was always there for everyone with his calm, heartfelt support.

Most of us enjoy friendships with many people, ranging from the casual to the deeply committed. Sometimes, however, we discover in a crisis that we have placed some of these people in the wrong column. Every cancer patient I have spoken with has had this experience. Some found that a person they had once counted on least now became their greatest strength. But others learned that, at this turning point in their lives, when a simple word of encouragement would have meant so much, there was silence or worse. Those people can pierce a heart.

Cancer is not just a disease. It is an event that can redefine a relationship. I began my battle with more friends than anyone had a right to have. I emerged with even more. To thank each would take more pages than I am allowed here, but it would be unconscionable to ignore them. They will always be in my prayers.

A few special people, however, stood by my side when it was the toughest, and when there was clearly no reward for doing so: Bob Turner, who time and time again was there when it counted; Dave Chatellier, the bravest man I ever met and the closest person to a brother that I will ever have; Dennis Hackin, the most caring person and loyal friend with whom anyone could ask to share a life (both are also cancer survivors); Lee Tawes, who stepped forward when the night was darkest; and Jay Coggan, who had no obligation at all and for whom there are no adequate words of thanks.

And finally, Skip Brittenham, Cliff Gilbert-Lurie and Jamey Cohen—who would tell you that they didn't do anything, but they did, and that modesty is part of what makes them truly special.

This book is deliberately short.

First, immediately after you've been diagnosed with cancer, your attention span shortens to the length of a gnat's blink. The days of wandering lazily through acres of prose in search of a nugget are gone. Time becomes something that lives and breathes, something that you never again take for granted.

Second, some of my own story is interesting, but since I'm not famous or someone of remarkable accomplishment, most of my own experience is best left on the cutting-room floor.

Third, parents are plenty smart already. They usually don't need three hundred pages of theory and footnotes to work something out with their kids, just a nudge in the right direction.

This book is not a medical or psychology text. I have had cancer twice, but I am not an expert in either the disease or in counseling people who have it. Those areas belong to doctors and other trained professionals. What I do have are graduate degrees in time logged in waiting rooms and the indignity of being poked, prodded, stuck, rolled over, photographed, cranked up and talked about like I wasn't there. I am a veteran at willing the phone to ring with the results of tests and lying awake at night in a cold sweat.

So now that I've told you that this book is short and without any medical value, what exactly is it?

Well, it's kind of a mixed bag. Partly the book is the personal story of someone whose closest brush with mortality before cancer was when he was nine and rode his bike down Suicide Hill with his eyes closed—someone who had taken his family, friends, career and good fortune largely for granted until he realized how fragile life is.

Another feature of the book is that I hope it will help you talk to your children about the cancer that has come into your life. For most of us, relating to our kids is not the first thing that leaps to mind when we hear the diagnosis. Later, when the thought finally does come, the prospect of sitting down with a ten-year-old and trying to make sense out of a disease that we barely understand ourselves is daunting.

Last, I hope the book will make those of you who have just joined this club—cancer patients who are also parents—realize that you have within yourself a great deal more resources than you ever imagined.

Twice I had to tell my children that I had cancer. Both times those conversations changed my life just as surely as the cancer did. I hope you have the same experience. Like it or not, you are never going to be the same person you were before cancer came. But sometimes, in our darkest moments, we can finally become the person we always wanted to be.

By the way, that whispering you hear on the wind is the rest of us praying for you.

NR

INTRODUCTION

Cancer is an equal opportunity disease.

Cancer doesn't care how many cars you have or what you do for a living. The disease is as likely to strike a man as a woman, a supermodel as a steelworker. The sick feeling in the pit of your stomach after being told that you have cancer isn't lessened by your income, your accomplishments or your job title.

Because cancer is so random, so arbitrary, so unconcerned whether you live in Beverly Hills or Harlem, it touches that little corner in each of our souls where we keep our most precious fears. War, famine and murder are, for most of us, distant and remote events. They arrive in our living rooms via the six o'clock news, and though we are appalled by their devastation, for the most part, we remain insulated from them.

Not cancer. Finding a person who has not known a friend, a family member, a coworker or a neighbor who has suffered from it is difficult. We have seen cancer change good lives forever, and many of us have lost to cancer people whom we can never replace. And what parent has not felt a strange bump on one of their children and uttered a silent prayer?

Few things are as traumatic as a cancer diagnosis. The moment the diagnosis is pronounced is often overwhelming. Though it is difficult to think of others when your own emotions are so raw and uncertain and your thoughts so personal, cancer has not happened to you alone. The diagnosis is now a member of your family—your whole family—and everybody who loves you will soon be right in there, struggling in their own way—especially your kids.

All of us dislike talking to our children about difficult things. We avoid it by telling ourselves that we are sparing them pain, which never works, because kids find out everything sooner or later. We may say that they won't understand, which is almost never the case, or we use the excuse that a professional should do the telling. Tell me someone—anyone—who knows more about your kids than you do.

No, the truth is that we usually just don't have a starting place, and we are deeply afraid of our emotions. Cancer is like that—a quiet terror. How do you speak rationally to the most important people in your life about something that makes you so angry that you want to lash out at everybody—even God? How do you talk to your kids—who often see you as invincible—about something that makes you so afraid that you want to curl up in bed and cry your eyes out?

How could anyone possibly understand how you feel—especially a kid? And besides, don't you have enough on your mind without having to try to explain all of this to anybody else? Shouldn't talking to your kids be something your husband or wife or mother or father can handle?

The answer is, sure, someone else can. But if you can summon the strength to do it yourself, you might find it one of the most fulfilling experiences of your life, one that creates a new strength and closeness between you and your children, and one that you will all carry with you for the rest of your lives. That happened to me, but it didn't start out that way.

I rank low on the touchy-feely scale. I run my own business, and I am used to being "In Charge." Most people who know me well describe me as reserved, self-confident and in control. People who do not like me as much would add the word *tough*. I have a difficult time asking anyone for anything; seeking moral support in a crisis would be unfathomable.

But when I was diagnosed with cancer the first time, I am not ashamed to say that I desperately wanted to talk to someone. Not a shoulder to cry on, but just an hour or two with someone sitting there and caring about what I said. Instead, I did what I have always done, what men are told to do from Day

One—I shut up, put my head down and got on with it.

The only problem was that I had these two kids: Andrew, who was thirteen at the time, and Trevor, eleven, who kept getting in the way of my being a tough guy. How was I supposed to fight on stoically, yet prepare them for what might not be a happy ending?

Worse, they were boys—the ones society expects will be the next generation of husbands, fathers, providers and protectors. Didn't I owe it to their future families to raise a couple of men who could handle themselves like, what else, men?

All of this meant that I had to talk to them. Not about the NFL, the NBA, how to throw a curveball or why we don't tell Grandma about the lizard living in the garage. But *real* talk, about things that men usually *never* talk about.

Frankly, this cancer business sucked. I now realized that I wasn't nearly as afraid of the doctors, the treatment, the pain or even the prospect of dying as I was of having to step out of character in front of my sons. I could pretend all I wanted, but if I wanted to do the right thing for my kids, I had to let them see me as a cancer patient, or as I would have described it at the time—"weak"—which was a long way from my carefully cultivated image of strong, invincible, infallible Dad.

I would like to say that once I came to this realization, I grabbed the bull and rode it: Sat those boys down, bared my soul and showed them what the insides of a real man looked like. That would be a lie. Instead I did what any floundering fool would do—I looked around for someone to do it for me.

Under the guise of seeking advice I spoke to my doctors, a researcher, a teacher, a minister, a priest and several close friends. After warming them up with a few questions about how I should talk to my kids about cancer, I kind of worked it into the conversation that I would really prefer to have someone do it for me. Someone smart and experienced. Someone who really understood these things better than

I did and could talk about them. Someone, well, like them, perhaps.

Nice try. "Sure, buddy, glad to help. Given any thought to growing a set lately? Maybe becoming a man? Doing it yourself?" That's not what they said, of course, but it was in their eyes.

Fresh out of ideas and surrogates, I remembered what a marine corps general once told me about landing on Guadalcanal as a young lieutenant. "The beach was mined, our own artillery was pounding us, my guys were shooting at anything that moved and I couldn't swim. Frankly, the enemy machine gun in front of me looked like the safest bet. Besides, I was sobbing, and I figured that if I got out in front, nobody would notice."

So exit John Wayne. Enter somebody I had not shaken hands with for a very long time— the Neil Russell who was afraid of the dark. That Neil Russell hadn't changed one bit, and I'd almost forgotten how much I hated him.

The New Age thing to say is that all of this was liberating—that in crisis I found myself, that I became more caring, more sensitive, more at peace. Maybe. You would have to ask somebody else about that. What I really found were my sons. I believe they found me, too.

I didn't really grasp the situation myself until a few weeks before I turned in this manuscript. When you read the Closing Note at the end of the book, you will understand.

One final thing. To those of you who have been wondering if there is a God: There is. I met him in the operating room.

CHAPTER ONE

To Parents: We Who Stumble and Bumble Our Way Through Things While Trying to Make It Look to Our Kids Like We Have a Plan

"You have cancer."

Twice in a little more than two years, I heard those three words—three words for which no one can ever prepare you. Once they are spoken to you or a loved one, nothing is ever the same again.

My grandmother used to say that every story has two beginnings—the one you choose to remember and the real one. You could never lie to her, because she would grill you until she discovered that real beginning.

My cancer story has two beginnings, too: the one I like to remember where I am the tough, hard-charging, I-will-beat-this-thing kind of guy, and the real one where I am not very tough at all. The second is less comfortable to tell, but the one on which my grandmother would have insisted.

3

When my assistant interrupted a conference in my office to tell me that my doctor wanted to speak to me, I asked the people with whom I was meeting to excuse me for a moment. I picked up the telephone.

I didn't know Dr. Solomon well, but I had been impressed with his quiet professionalism and easy smile when my regular physician, Dr. Goodman, first sent me to him. A no-nonsense straight-talker, he apologized for interrupting my meeting and went directly to the point.

"The results of the precautionary tests I ordered last week have just been faxed to me," he said. Then he paused. I had seen enough medical shows to know that nothing good comes after a pause, and I was right. "You have cancer," he said evenly. And there was more. The tests were imprecise with respect to the cancer's exact location, and knowing whether or not it had metastasized—migrated elsewhere—was impossible. In addition, the cancer had graded out "hot," meaning that I had an aggressive form of the disease.

I was married to Sandi, the girl I used to tease in high school, and we had two healthy young sons, Andrew, thirteen, and Trevor, eleven. I had my dream job as president of a television and motion picture production company and was lucky enough to be able to work with some of Hollywood's best talent. I was also fit, ran twenty-five miles a week, ate properly and didn't smoke. Until that moment, my biggest problem was that the Little League team I was coaching had both the highest batting average and the worst win/loss record in our division—an anomaly several parents had begun to attribute to management. Otherwise, I was having a pretty good life.

I didn't tell anyone about my diagnosis right away. I am by nature a deliberate person, and I wanted to be sure that I understood as many of the ramifications of the disease and the potential courses of action before I began trying to explain anything to anyone else. I also needed to complete a series of more sophisticated medical tests, and I wanted to do that without alarming anyone in my family.

During that first week, I did what we are all taught to do—I vacuumed up every available scrap of information about cancer from my doctor, the library and the Internet. I also spoke to physicians and researchers at Johns Hopkins, Memorial Sloan-Kettering and the Mayo Clinic for information on the latest techniques in treating my particular form of cancer. It's amazing who you can get on the telephone and what you can convince them to tell you when you are really motivated. (It also didn't hurt that I produced movies for a living.)

Finally, with at least a working knowledge of the disease and the options available to me, I put my sons to bed, poured a couple of glasses of red wine and broke the news to my wife.

All things considered, she took it pretty well. She had some questions, of course, but fewer than I had expected. And so, wine glasses raised, we began a new phase of our marriage: the cancer phase.

Looking back, it now seems unfathomable that I could have gone so far without once considering how I was going to tell Andrew and Trevor that I was sick. I had been so focused on satisfying my own thirst for knowledge that it truly never crossed my mind that they were also involved.

Now, I was guilty of giving my sons the same short shrift that adults routinely give children when life-altering events occur. *After all, they're "just kids," aren't they? How could they understand something as complex and terrifying as losing your job ... or going to war ... or cancer?*

But kids are family members, too, the ones who don't have years of accumulated wisdom and experience to fall back on in a crisis, and the ones who never seem to have a vote on important issues. As I sat there drinking wine with my wife, I began to realize that telling my sons about cancer was, perhaps, the most important responsibility I had yet faced as a parent. Moreover, the way I handled it would be something they *and* I would remember for the rest of our lives. Added to that thought was the terrifying realization that I didn't have a clue where to start.

So I went back into research mode: back to the library, back to the doctors and back to the Internet. A week earlier I had been able to access reams of data about cancer treatments so cutting-edge that news of them had not yet reached my physicians, but this time I came up mostly empty.

I did find some older books that talked peripherally about kids and cancer as well as a considerable body of work on grief counseling. But when it came to a simple, straightforward book about the state of cancer at the dawn of the twenty-first century that my sons and I could sit down and read together, the literature was not just thin, it was nonexistent.

So, for lack of a better way to approach the problem, I went to my word processor and tried to think like a kid. It wasn't scientific, but based on my observations as a father and baseball coach, I knew that kids can usually comprehend just about anything, if you give it to them straight and in terms that they understand.

From experience I also knew that, when talking to kids, the deadliest phrase in the English language is, "Anybody got any questions?" Almost nobody thinks in terms of what he or she doesn't know, especially a child. Conversely, I had discovered that if I asked my baseball team a simple, direct question like, "What's our bunt sign?" I might get thirteen different answers, but I would immediately know who needed help.

With these rather basic precepts in mind, I typed out a series of questions about cancer, the same questions I had wanted answered when I first learned that I had the disease. Then I went back and answered each question—simply—using language a child might use to explain the rules of a game to a new playmate.

A few days later, brimming with information, I closed the family room door, opened three Cokes and tried not to appear too nervous. But looking into my sons' young faces, my palms turned sweaty and my mouth went dry. *Was I about to give them too much information?*

Not enough? Were my explanations going to be too technical? Or perhaps condescending? Should I even be doing this? Pushing back the doubt, I swallowed hard and began.

To my surprise, after a rocky first few moments, things started to come together. A few tears came, and for a brief moment I longed to be aboard the Orient Express bound for Istanbul, but then things leveled off.

When I finished, a long pause ensued before anybody said anything. Then Trevor, my youngest son, looked into my eyes with more intensity than I could have imagined he possessed and asked a question I could never have anticipated, "Daddy, can I still kiss you?"

It was so simple, yet so profound and so moving that it was a long moment before I could answer him. When I finally answered, "Yes, you can," it was like a relief valve had been opened for all of us, and for the next hour we engaged in one of the most intelligent, most touching discussions we had ever had. None of us will ever forget it.

A little over two years later, when my cancer returned, my sons and I sat down with a new series of questions, but this time things were different. By now, I had met dozens of parents who had had to tell their sons and daughters about cancer, and Andrew and Trevor had found that many of their school friends had dealt with the same fears that they had. My sons were older now as well, and their questions were much more insightful and profound. This time we talked a lot longer than an hour, not just about the pain that cancer brings to a family, but about the strength that can come from the experience as well.

I wish I had never had cancer. No one deserves this horrible disease. You can't really explain to anyone but another cancer patient how it changes you, and the fear it leaves in the pit of your stomach never truly goes away. I can honestly say, however, that as close as my sons and I had been before, cancer brought us closer, and for that I owe it a debt.

Having compiled all of this kid intelligence,

just throwing it in a drawer seemed such a waste. So, in the hope that it might help someone else, I wrote down what Andrew, Trevor and I had learned. Then I gave everything to Neil Barth, M.D., a highly respected oncologist, and Dr. Margaret Reedy, a clinical psychologist friend who works with families in crisis. I asked each of them to review and correct what I had written. Remarkably, they made very few changes, and the result is the book you are holding.

The chapter divisions are self-explanatory. As you begin each new chapter, I would encourage you to review with your child the material that you have already covered. Children find comfort in going over information that they already know, and after they have lived with cancer for a while, some of their earlier questions will become much more personal.

In closing, I would like to make four comments:

First, as I have previously said, this book is not a medical text but instead presents questions and answers with which to begin a conversation about cancer with your child. By design the presentation is simple and general. Only a medical practitioner can provide specific information about any disease, and one should look to those dedicated men and women for detailed answers about cancer.

Second, remember that kids are smart, and though they might sometimes pose questions that are difficult or uncomfortable to answer, the truth is always preferable to a diversion. By the same token, younger children need less detailed, simpler explanations while older ones can understand and process more complex information. Also, check back with your kids from time to time, both to let them know that you have not forgotten them as well as for periodic updates on topics or aspects of your disease that might be bothering them.

Third, cancer is intensely personal, and no one, not even someone suffering from it, can adequately describe its effect on another. Similarly, no two individuals respond to the same type of cancer in exactly the same way. So some of the following material may not apply to another person's experience with the disease. In an effort to accommodate those differences, I have intentionally left blanks in some of the answers for moms and dads to discuss their specific experiences.

Last, please tell your kids that sometimes even well-meaning people make insensitive remarks—statements that might not be accurate or that are based on rumor or speculation. Cancer is a big event that will start a gossip's tongue wagging faster than a local sighting of the Publishers Clearing House Prize Patrol. Whatever your kids hear outside the home, they should either ignore it or bring it to you so that you can set them straight.

I apologize in advance to anyone who feels that this book goes either too far or not far enough. The effort is truly my best.

CHAPTER TWO

To Kids: Those Whom We Cannot Imagine Our Lives Without

Cancer is a scary word. I know because I've had cancer twice. It's a word that grown-ups sometimes whisper around children. But whispering won't make cancer go away, and whispering won't make kids any less afraid.

When my doctor told me that I had cancer the first time, one of the first things I thought about was how I was going to tell my two sons, Trevor and Andrew.

Trevor, my youngest son, was in sixth grade and was a happy, smiling kid who loved making people laugh. He played quarterback on his football team, loved video games and had a million friends. His favorite television show was *Saved by the Bell,* his favorite food was mushroom pizza and his favorite drink was chocolate milk—which he made using so much syrup that the milk always ended up looking like brown goo.

Trevor collected all kinds of sports stuff, and his prized possession was a Mickey Mantle autographed baseball. On Saturday mornings, he and I would wake up before everybody else and sit together on the sofa, watching movies like *Star Wars,* and every night before bed, I would read him an adventure story.

My other son, Andrew, was an extremely quiet boy. When he was very little, his favorite game was hide-and-seek, and he would find a really good hiding place then sit absolutely still. Sometimes nobody could find him, and we would just have to wait until he came out. Once, he stayed hidden for so long that we were afraid something had happened to him. We were just getting ready to call the police when he showed up, smiling. He had been hiding beneath a covered chair right under our noses the whole time. We were upset that he had scared us so much, but we were so busy hugging him that pretty soon we forgot to be angry.

Andrew was in eighth grade when I got sick. He was an all-star pitcher in Little League and a very good student. He collected all kinds of things from flags of countries to baseball cards, and he had an amazing ability to memorize things. For example, he knew the license plate number of every car in the neighborhood, dozens of them. It was kind of spooky, because he even remembered the names of every student in every class he had ever been in, all the way back to kindergarten. Andrew's two favorite things to do were to play catch and to have me read to him. I did both every chance I had.

I loved Andrew and Trevor more than anything in my life, and I didn't want them to be afraid. But I knew that I had an obligation to tell them about the cancer I had. So one day, the three of us opened some Cokes and sat down with some questions I had written and started talking.

The experience was amazing. Yes, my sons were scared, but they were also curious. They wanted to know everything about cancer, and even though I thought I had prepared for our conversation, I found out that they had a lot more questions than I could answer.

Two years after I got cancer the first time, it came back. As I once again faced talking to my sons about my disease, I began thinking about how many other moms and dads find out they have cancer. I thought that maybe it would help some of them to be able to talk to their kids about their disease, and for their kids to understand it a little better, if they had a book to read together.

So, as I entered my second round of cancer treatments, I began writing down some of the questions that people told me that their kids had asked when they had talked about cancer. At the same time, Andrew and Trevor interviewed friends of theirs whose fathers or mothers had been diagnosed with cancer. They also went on the Internet and found other kids who were dealing with a parent with cancer and asked them what they wanted to know most. The result is this book.

I hope it helps.

To help parents and children talk or communicate with each other, I have left space after each question so that you can write down your own thoughts and notes as you go. This process personalizes the questions for better discussion and provides a time capsule at an important time in the family's history. Feel free to use these pages however you want. Write in them, draw pictures in the margins and make the book *yours.*

But before you begin, I would like you to stop for a moment and just give each other a hug and a kiss. Doctors can do lots of things for cancer, but nothing feels as good as the warm touch of someone you love.

CHAPTER THREE

A Cancer Diagnosis:
Can I Still Kiss You?

Q. What is cancer?

A. *Your body, my body . . . all living things . . . are made up of tiny objects called cells. Cells are a little bit like Legos. Bunches of them fit together in just the right way to form different parts of the body. Some bunches of cells become skin, like the skin on your arms; some become organs, like your heart; and some become bone, like the ones in your legs. Once in a while, a few of these cells can get sick, and they make the cells around them sick, too. The sick cells are called cancer.*

Q. What makes the cells get sick?

A. *No one knows exactly how or why it happens. There seem to be different causes for different kinds of cancer, and scientists are working hard to find out what each of them is.*

Q. Does everybody get cancer?

A. *No, some people do, and some people don't. But the risk for cancer goes up when people do certain things, like smoke cigarettes.*

Q. Why did *you* have to get it? Did you do something wrong?

A. *My doctor told me:*

_____

_____

_____

_____

_____

_____

Q. Can kids get cancer, too?

A. *Children don't get cancer as often as adults do, but sometimes it does happen. When it does, doctors work very hard to make them well, just like they do with adults. Do you know any children who have had cancer?*

Q. Did you catch cancer from me?

A. *Absolutely not.*

Q. Can I catch it from you?

A. *No, cancer is not contagious. Each person gets cancer on their own.*

Q. Can our dog or my goldfish get cancer?

A. *Yes, people, animals . . . even trees . . . can get cancer. Anything made of cells can.*

Q. Can the doctor give you a shot to make you better?

A. *Sometimes doctors give people who have cancer special kinds of medicine through a needle, but there isn't one simple shot to cure cancer, yet. The good news is that new medicines are being discovered all the time.*

Q. Can the doctor give me a shot to keep me from getting cancer?

A. *No, that kind of shot does not exist, and because there are so many different types of cancer, finding one medicine that would prevent all kinds is unlikely. However, scientists are learning more about cancer than ever before, and they are now working to develop tests and medicines that will target certain kinds of cancer before they get out of control. So early detection is still the most important factor in cancer treatment.*

Q. How does somebody find out that they have cancer?

A. *Sometimes a person feels sick in a way he or she has never been sick before or notices something different about his or her body, like bleeding where there shouldn't be any blood or a cough or some spot or lump on their body that won't go away. And sometimes, the doctor finds something wrong during a regular checkup.*

Q. How did you find out you had cancer?

A. *I found out when* _____

_____

_____

_____

_____

_____.

Q. Why didn't you tell us you were feeling sick?

A. *I didn't tell you because* _____

_____

_____

_____

_____

_____.

Q. Does cancer hurt?

A. *Sometimes it does, but often there is no pain at all. That is why it is important for doctors to conduct tests.*

Q. Does your cancer hurt? Does it hurt a lot?

A. My cancer _____

_____

_____

_____

_____

_____.

Q. Do you cry when it hurts?

A. Yes, sometimes I do, but most of the time when adults with cancer cry, it's not because of the pain. It's because they're sad or tired or just feel overwhelmed. Have you ever seen a grown-up cry? How did it make you feel?

Q. Do people die from having cancer?

A. *Unfortunately, some people do. But others are treated successfully. Those people can then lead normal, happy lives.*

Q. Are you going to die?

A. *The doctors are going to do everything they can to make me well again, but sometimes things can happen that no one wants or expects.*

Q. Are you afraid of dying?

A. *Yes, I am. Death is a scary thing to think about, and it's okay for you to be scared, too. Let's agree that we'll talk about it whenever it's bothering you. In the meantime, let's try to be hopeful and optimistic.*

Q. What will happen to me if you die?

A. *It will be a difficult time, but we have a very strong family, all of whom love you very much. If I do die, they will be there to take care of you.*

Q. I will be so lonely if you die.

A. *I know, but that is a natural reaction when we lose someone we love. But I will always be there in your memories.*

Q. If you die, will I get a new dad?

A. *I will always be your dad.*

Q. What if Mom gets cancer, too?

A. *Chances are she won't, but if she does, the doctors will try hard to make her well, too.*

Q. If you both die, who will take care of me?

A. *That's probably not going to happen. It's more likely that we'll be here to nag you about cleaning your room. But Mom and I have talked about it, and this is what would happen to you:*

_____

_____

_____.

(Note to parents: *The things that kids are most concerned about are: Who will take care of me? Will I have to move away? Will I still be able to live with my brothers and sisters? Will I be able to keep my dog? And what will happen if my new caregiver dies, too?*)

Q. I'm just a kid. What can I do to help you get better?

A. *You can love me, and you can include me in your prayers.*

Q. Can God make your cancer go away?

A. *God and doctors working together make a very powerful team.*

Q. Will you still be able to hold me when I'm scared?

A. *Yes, and it's okay to be afraid. It's also okay to ask questions, even the scary ones. Is there anything you would like to ask me now? You can say anything you want, even if it's not very nice.*

Q. Is it all right to be angry?

A. *Yes, it is, and it's also okay to cry. But it's also important to talk to someone when you feel angry or sad. It's never good to keep those feelings bottled up inside. You and I are going to talk a lot about cancer, but it's also okay to talk to a teacher or a relative or someone else that you trust. Can you think of someone you would feel comfortable talking to?*

(Note to parents: *It would be a good idea to contact that person ahead of time so that they will be aware of the situation.*)

Q. Can I tell my friends about your cancer?

A. *Yes, but it's important to understand that you will probably know more about cancer than your friends do, so it might be a good idea if I had a conversation with their parents first to explain the situation. That way your friends will have somebody to talk to if they have questions. Okay? By the way, do you know if any of your friends' parents have had cancer?*

Q. Is there anybody else I can talk to?

A. *Absolutely. Talking about things that are bothering you is helpful and healthy. Sometimes a teacher, a minister, a rabbi, a coach or even another parent can be a good person to seek out. Let's make a list of some of the people you think you would be comfortable talking to:*

_____

_____

_____

_____

_____

_____

Q. Can I still kiss you?

A. *As much as you want, with a few extras thrown in.*

Now it's your chance as parents and children to write some questions and answers of your own about the diagnosis of cancer.

KIDS

If you have any other questions about the diagnosis of cancer, write them here:

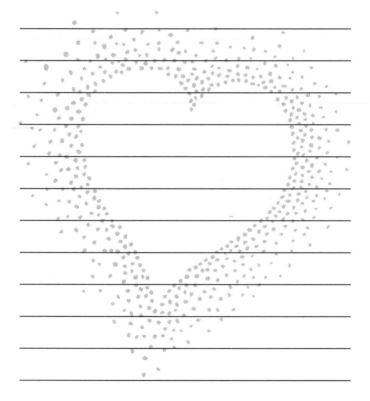

READER/CUSTOMER CARE SURVEY

We care about your opinions. Please take a moment to fill out this Reader Survey card and mail it back to us. As a special "thank you" we'll send you exciting news about interesting books and a valuable **Gift Certificate.**

Please PRINT using ALL CAPS

First Name _____ MI. ___ Last Name _____

Address _____ City _____

ST ___ Zip _____ Email: _____

Phone # (___) _____ Fax # (___) _____

(1) Gender:

_____ Female _____ Male

(2) Age:

_____ 12 or under _____ 40-59
_____ 13-19 _____ 60+
_____ 20-39

(3) What attracts you most to a book?

(Please rank 1-4 in order of preference.)

	1	2	3	4
3) Title	○	○	○	○
4) Cover Design	○	○	○	○
5) Author	○	○	○	○
6) Content	○	○	○	○

(7) Where do you usually buy books?

*Please fill in your top **TWO** choices.*

1) _____ Bookstore
2) _____ Religious Bookstore
3) _____ Online
4) _____ Book Club/Mail Order
5) _____ Price Club (Costco, Sam's Club, etc.)
6) _____ Retail Store (Target, Wal-Mart, etc.)

Comments:

_____
_____
_____
_____
_____
_____

BUSINESS REPLY MAIL

FIRST-CLASS MAIL PERMIT NO 45 DEERFIELD BEACH, FL

POSTAGE WILL BE PAID BY ADDRESSEE

HEALTH COMMUNICATIONS, INC.

3201 SW 15TH STREET

DEERFIELD BEACH FL 33442-9875

PARENTS

If there's anything else you want your kids to know about your diagnosis of cancer, write it here:

_____

_____

_____

_____

_____

_____

_____

_____

_____

_____

_____

_____

_____

Love

Laugh

Hope

Encourage

Heal

Pray

Live

CHAPTER FOUR

Surgery: When Hands Become Magic

Q. What is surgery?

A. A special doctor called a surgeon, who went to school for a long time to learn how to remove cancer from people, will put me into the hospital and cut the cancer out of me with a very sharp knife. The process of cutting it out is called surgery, and the knife the surgeon uses is called a scalpel.

Q. Will it hurt?

A. No, I won't feel anything during the surgery. Another doctor called an anesthesiologist will give me some medicine called an anesthetic that will put me to sleep. Afterward, while I'm healing, I may have some pain, but the doctor can give me medicine that will help me not feel it.

Q. How long will you be asleep during surgery?

A. *That will depend upon how long the surgeon will need to remove the cancer.*

Q. How do they put you back together after the surgery?

A. *The surgeon will use a very fine needle and thread or metal clips like staples to hold the skin together until it heals. I know it sounds painful, but it really isn't.*

Q. If I bump into you by mistake, will it mess everything up, or will it just hurt?

A. *It would probably just hurt, but just to be on the safe side, in the beginning, we need to be really careful. Then in a few days, I should be healed enough so that we can stop worrying so much.*

Q. After the surgery, will the cancer be gone so you can come home?

A. *I'll be able to come home after a while, but the doctor won't know if the cancer is gone until some tests are performed later.*

Q. What happens if it isn't gone?

A. *Then the doctor may have to do some other things to try to make it go away.*

Q. What other things?

A. *Maybe more surgery, or radiation treatments or chemotherapy.*

Now it's your chance as parents and children to write some questions and answers of your own about surgery.

KIDS

If you have any other questions about surgery, write them here:

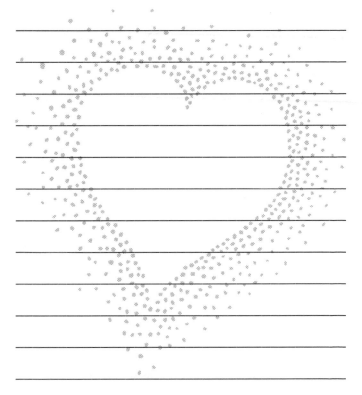

PARENTS

If there's anything else you want your kids to know about surgery or if there's something you want to look up together later, write it here:

_____

_____

_____

_____

_____

_____

_____

_____

_____

_____

_____

_____

_____

Love

Laugh

Hope

Encourage

Heal

Pray

Live

CHAPTER FIVE

Radiation:
Invisible Rays That Heal

Q. Radiation? What's that?

A. *Radiation is a little difficult to explain, but a specially trained doctor called a radiation oncologist uses invisible rays to attack cancer cells and kill them. An oncologist is a cancer doctor.*

Q. Invisible rays?

A. *Yes, think about the wind for a minute. When the wind is blowing, you can't actually see it, but you know it's there because you can feel it on your face, can't you? So the wind is real, but it's invisible. Doctors have very special kinds of medicine that emit invisible rays that kill cancer cells. Like the wind, you can't see these rays, but they're real.*

Q. How do they get the rays into the cancer to kill it?

A. *In two very different ways. The first is to use a very large, very complicated machine called an accelerator to aim the rays at the place in the body where the cancer is growing. The second way is to use a tube, a needle or surgery to place the medicine that emits the rays directly into the area of the body where the cancer is growing.*

Q. What are they going to do to you?

A. *They will* _____

_____

_____

_____

_____

_____.

Q. Where do they keep the accelerator machine?

A. At a place called a cancer treatment center. Most treatment centers are connected to hospitals, but some are in office buildings. People with cancer go there to be treated.

Q. Does a doctor use the machine on you?

A. In the beginning, a doctor will set up my treatment schedule, determine how much radiation I need and where it will be applied to my body. Then, specially trained people called radiation therapists will take over and treat me.

Q. Radiation therapists?

A. Radiation therapists and the people who give chemotherapy are the heroes of cancer treatment. They are the people the patient sees every day to be treated, and sometimes the patients and these therapists become friends for life.

Q. How long do the radiation treatments last?

A. *Each radiation treatment only takes a few minutes, but I need one every day, for several weeks. I'll get the weekends off to rest.*

Q. Why can't the therapist just give the treatments all at once and make you better right away?

A. *That would be nice, but the rays don't work that way. They're too powerful and would hurt the good cells, too. It's a little like studying math. No one can learn everything about math in one day, but if you learn a little bit each day, pretty soon you know everything in the book. Sometimes slower is better.*

Q. What does the room look like where they keep the machine?

A. *It's very clean and quiet with soft lighting. There is a bed in the middle of the room, and the machine is over the bed. Some people give their room and their machine nicknames. One man named his room "Mission Control" and his machine "E.T." Can you help me think up a name for my room and machine?*

Q. Can I see the room and the machine?

A. *Absolutely. You can visit and you can also meet the therapists.*

Q. Does the machine make a lot of noise?

A. *No, the electric motor that moves it around sounds a little bit like an air conditioner starting up. When the machine is actually operating, though, it's pretty quiet, except for some soft clicks and buzzes.*

Q. Do you have to get undressed?

A. *Yes, and I have to have some marks drawn on my skin to show the therapists where to aim the radiation. The marks are made with different colored Magic Markers. They're just like the ones you use in school. So for a while I'm going to look like somebody drew maps on me.*

Q. Can you feel the rays coming out of the machine like I can feel the wind?

A. *No, I can't feel anything, but as the treatments continue, the skin over the treatment area will probably become red like a sunburn.*

Q. Won't that hurt?

A. *Yes, but if I'm careful, I'll still be able to do most of the things I normally do. You'll have to try not to bump into me, though.*

Q. Will you still be able to go to my soccer games?

A. *I'm really going to try, but sometimes I might be tired or in some pain, and it will be difficult for me to go out. But I'll make you a deal. I'll go to every game I can, and when I'm not able to, you and I will sit down afterward, and you'll tell me everything that happened. Deal?*

Now it's your chance as parents and children to write some questions and answers of your own about radiation.

KIDS

If you have any other questions about radiation, write them here:

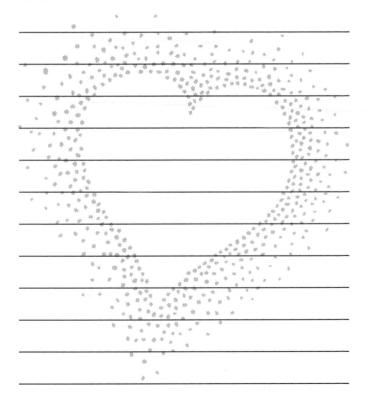

PARENTS

If there's anything else you want your kids to know about radiation, or if there's something you want to look up together later, write it here:

_____

_____

_____

_____

_____

_____

_____

_____

_____

_____

_____

_____

Love

Laugh

Hope

Encourage

Heal

Pray

Live

CHAPTER SIX

Chemotherapy:
If Medicine Is Good,
Why Does It Make
You Sick?

Q. What is chemotherapy?

A. *Chemotherapy is a medical treatment where cancer-killing medicine is put into a patient's bloodstream.*

Q. Do they use a needle to give you the medicine?

A. *Yes. Sometimes chemotherapy medicine is given in a pill, but most of the time, it is given through a needle in either the hand or the arm.*

Q. Why do they put it in your hand or your arm if that's not where the cancer is?

A. *Because blood travels to all parts of the body, the doctors will use my bloodstream to get the cancer-killing medicine to the cancer cells wherever they are. The veins in the hand and arm are close to the surface and easier to work with. Can you show me one of your veins?*

Q. Will chemotherapy make you well?

A. *No one knows for sure, but it is the best treatment available for my cancer, and my doctor is very good. Everybody, including me, is going to do the best they can.*

Q. Where do you get chemotherapy?

A. *At either a hospital, a doctor's office or a cancer treatment center.*

Q. How many times do you have to go for chemotherapy?

A. *In my case,* _____

_____

_____

_____

_____

_____.

Q. Then will you be better?

A. Not at first, and this is difficult to explain, but the medicine they use in chemotherapy is very powerful and can have other effects on the body. I may get sick to my stomach and lose some of my hair. The medicine will be attacking the cancer, but it will probably also make me very tired, and it is also possible that I will lose some weight and be too weak to do some things.

Q. You're already sick. Why do you have to do something that will make you even sicker?

A. I know this is difficult. It's a hard time for all of us, but especially for you. It's scary when a mom or dad gets sick, but chemotherapy is my best chance to kill the cancer so I can get back to being with you all of the time. Sometimes you may just want to cry. If you do, it's okay, but let's agree that you'll always tell me if something is bothering you, even if it seems silly. Okay?

Q. How will the doctors know the chemotherapy is working?

A. *Through regular tests on my blood and with X rays and something called a CAT scan.*

Q. Can I be with you while you get your chemotherapy?

A. *I will talk to the doctor and arrange for you to visit the treatment room and meet the people who are going to be treating me. However, it isn't possible for you to be there when I'm receiving the medicine.*

Q. Why not?

A. *The medicine I will be receiving is very strong, and people who are not being treated should not be exposed to it. This is especially true for children. There is also another reason, and this may be difficult for you to understand, but fighting cancer is very personal and this is one of the times when I need to be alone with my doctors.*

Q. Will the chemotherapy hurt you?

A. *Sometimes chemotherapy can cause other types of problems, but that doesn't happen very often. The doctors and nurses will be watching me carefully.*

Q. What can I do to help?

A. *You can help around the house and try to avoid fighting with your brothers and sisters, but I don't want you to stop being a kid. Even though this is not an easy time for our family, we are still going to have as much fun as possible.*

Q. Can I pray for you?

A. *I would like that.*

Now it's your chance as parents and children to write some questions and answers of your own about chemotherapy.

KIDS

If you have any other questions about chemotherapy treatment write them here:

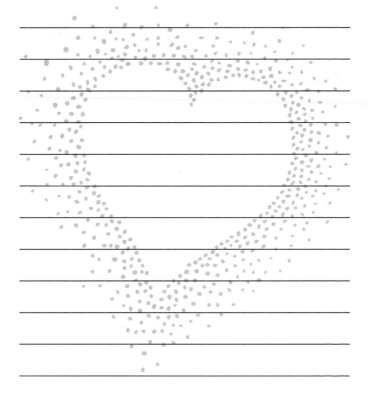

_____

_____

_____

_____

_____

_____

_____

_____

_____

_____

_____

_____

PARENTS

If there's anything else you want your kids to know about chemotherapy, or if there's something you want to look up together later, write it here:

_____

_____

_____

_____

_____

_____

_____

_____

_____

_____

_____

Love

Laugh

Hope

Encourage

Heal

Pray

Live

CHAPTER SEVEN

During Treatment: Why Can't You Be Like You Used to Be?

Q. Why are you angry with me so often?

A. *I'm not angry with you, Sweetheart. Sometimes I don't feel very well, and I overreact to things that I would normally ignore. I promise you that I will work as hard as I can to do better. You can help by reminding me when I forget and by forgiving me when I slip up.*

Q. Have you and Mom stopped loving each other because you have cancer?

A. *Absolutely not. Not all people deal with cancer the same way, and even though it might sometimes seem like Mom and I are different, she and I still love each other very much. We're the same people we were before I got cancer.*

Q. Then why is Mom always so angry? I don't like it.

A. *Mom loves all of us very much, and sometimes it's difficult seeing the people you love get sick. Let's talk to her about it, but let's try to be understanding, too, okay?*

Q. I don't like being around sick people.

A. *That makes two of us, but sometimes it just can't be helped. Getting through tough times is part of what makes a family strong. It also helps us really appreciate the good times.*

Q. Sometimes I have trouble sleeping and get bad dreams.

A. *Those are natural reactions when we are worried. I have bad dreams, too. Usually it gets better as time passes, but we need to talk about it. What kind of dreams are you having?*

Q. I hate the people who are hurting you.

A. *Sometimes in medicine, people have to hurt people to help them. When you get a cut, we have to clean it before we bandage it, don't we? Cleaning a cut sometimes hurts, but you understand that we're just making sure the cut heals properly. Treating cancer is the same thing. The doctors, nurses and therapists are working hard to make me well again, but in the process they might have to hurt me. They don't want to, but sometimes it can't be avoided. Let's try to focus on the good that they're doing.*

Q. But you don't seem to be getting better. You seem to be getting worse.

A. *In a way, that's true, but unfortunately that's the way chemotherapy works. In time, things will get better.*

Q. I don't like the way you look. You're skinny and you're almost bald.

A. *I'll admit that I've looked better, but as soon as the chemotherapy is over, hopefully I'll start to look like myself again.*

Q. One of my friends said that you look like a freak.

A. *You can't do anything about that, except learn from it. Sometimes when a person looks different, it makes other people uncomfortable, and they say things that can hurt. Do you know anyone who looks different? How do you treat them?*

Q. Somebody said that they could catch cancer from me.

A. *You know that isn't true, so what did you tell them?*

Q. I want to sit on your lap, but I can't.

A. *I would love to be able to hold you, Darling, and I promise that just as soon as I can, we will hug until you get tired of it.*

Q. I feel guilty that I can go out and play, and you have to stay in the house so much.

A. *Please don't feel guilty. Run and play and have as much fun as possible. It makes me feel good when I know you're doing the things that kids are supposed to do. Because when I'm better, we're going to have so much fun together that you'll beg me to stop.*

Q. When are you going to go back to work? I'm afraid we're going to run out of money.

A. *We'll get by. The most important thing right now is for me to get well so that I can go back to work and not have to worry about the cancer anymore. Then, all of our lives can start getting back to normal.*

Q. Why don't you eat with the rest of the family?

A. *Sometimes I don't feel well enough to join you at mealtimes, and sometimes I don't like the smell of food, even foods I like. I've got an idea, though. Let's spread a blanket on the floor of the bedroom one night after dinner, and everybody can come in and have milk and cookies and talk. What kind of cookies should we get?*

Q. All you ever seem to do is sleep.

A. *I know. It's no fun, is it? The good news is that all that sleep is helping my body regenerate itself from the cancer treatments. Just as soon as I'm better, my plan is to order a big pizza for us and then stay up late watching television.*

Q. Cancer always seems to come first in our house. I hate cancer!

A. *You're right. We do spend a lot of time talking about cancer. Let's fix that. Here's what we'll do. Every member of the family is responsible for finding a good story to tell tomorrow night. It can be from a book, a magazine, a newspaper or something that happened to you or your imagination. Then we're going to spread out the blanket in the bedroom, get our milk and cookies and tell our stories. The one with the best story gets a prize. You're in charge of picking the prizes.*

Q. I've heard you talk about a support group. What's a support group, and why do you need to go to it?

A. *Sometimes a group of people who have the same problem, like cancer, feel better when they meet together and talk about it. They can exchange information and gain strength from one another. It's a way to help people who are struggling with their cancer and, at the same time, help yourself as well. In some ways, it's like a bunch of students who are all having trouble with math. Chances are they each know something that the others don't, and by getting together and sharing information, they can help everybody pass the test.*

Q. Is there a support group for kids? Can I go to one?

A. *You certainly may. I will ask my doctors what they recommend.*

(Note to parents: *You may also want to check some of the resources listed at the end of the book.*)

Now it's your chance as parents and children to write some questions and answers of your own about the way cancer patients act during treatment.

KIDS

If you have any other questions about how your parent is acting while they're undergoing treatment for cancer, write them here:

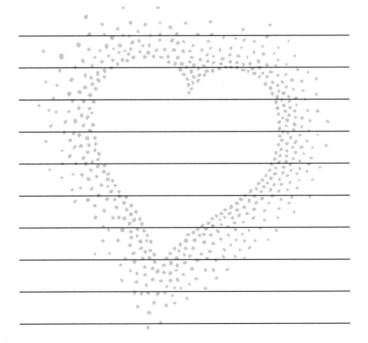

_____

_____

_____

_____

_____

_____

_____

_____

PARENTS

If there's anything else you want your kids to know about the way you're acting while undergoing treatment for cancer, or if there's something you want to look up together later, write it here:

_____

_____

_____

_____

_____

_____

_____

_____

_____

_____

_____

_____

Love

Laugh

Hope

Encourage

Heal

Pray

Live

CHAPTER EIGHT

The Future:
Making Every Day
the Best It Can
Possibly Be

Q. Will your cancer come back?

A. *No one knows for sure. There is always the chance that it will, but the doctors are going to be watching me very closely.*

Q. If it comes back, what will happen?

A. *I'll have to be treated again.*

Q. I don't want that to happen!

A. *Neither do I, but we have to be on the lookout just in case. In the meantime, let's make it a point to enjoy as many things as we can. How about choosing something special for dinner tomorrow night?*

Q. Do you still have to go back to the hospital?

A. *Not like before, but I will have to have regular checkups.*

Q. Can you do something to keep the cancer away?

A. *The best thing I can do is live as healthy a lifestyle as possible and see my doctor regularly.*

Q. You're different now. I want you to be like you were before.

A. *Often people who have a traumatic experience in their lives change a little bit because of it. I know one way I've changed. Now I _____*

_____

_____. How do you think I've changed? _____

_____.

Do you think you have changed since I got cancer? How? _____

_____

_____.

Q. I don't like any of the changes.

A. *I know, but sometimes if you give yourself a chance to get used to new things, you find out they're not so bad after all. So why don't we give the new me a little time and see what happens? But let's agree that if something is bothering you, we'll discuss it, and if I can make things better, I will.*

Q. I wake up in the night, and I'm scared.

A. *This has been a very difficult ordeal for all of us. The next time you get scared in the night, please come and get me so we can talk . . . no matter what time it is. Promise?*

Q. When I get older, will I get cancer because you did?

A. *When a mom or dad gets cancer, it doesn't mean that their children will get it, too. For certain kinds of cancer, however, the children of parents with that type of cancer could be at increased risk and should be checked regularly. Finding cancer early is still one of the best weapons for treating it.*

Q. Cancer has been the worst thing that ever happened to our family.

A. *I wish I had never gotten cancer, and I wish our family had never had to deal with it, but something good has come of it, too. It has helped me understand what is really important in life. I love you very, very much. Can you think of anything in your life that is better since I got sick?*

Now it's your chance as parents and children to write some questions and answers of your own about the future.

KIDS

If you have any other questions about the future, write them here:

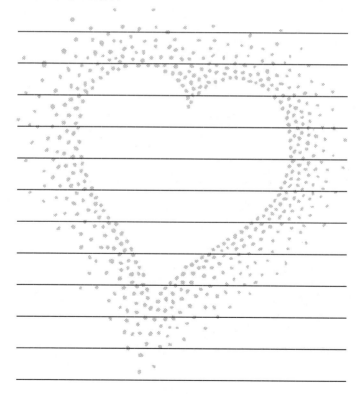

PARENTS

If there's anything else you want your kids to know about the future, or if there's something you want to look up together later, write it here:

_____

_____

_____

_____

_____

_____

_____

_____

_____

_____

_____

_____

_____

Love

Laugh

Hope

Encourage

Heal

Pray

Live

CHAPTER NINE

Your Questions and Thoughts: The Specialness of You

The following section is for you and your children to write down questions that come to you in the course of talking about cancer. Answering some of them might require that you do additional research together, but that can be another way of communicating during a difficult time.

If you find yourself having trouble getting started, you might encourage your children to write make-believe letters to someone they feel close to—you, a friend, a teacher, a relative or, if it is consistent with your family's beliefs, God or some other Higher Power. In their letters, they can describe their fears and ask the questions that they want answers to most.

Afterward, you can sit down together and transfer their thoughts into this book. I can assure you that you will find out things about

your children that you never would otherwise—
and you will both be moved.

?_____

_____

?_____

_____

?_____

_____

?_____

_____

?_____

_____

?_____

_____

?_____

_____

?_____

_____

?_____

_____

?_____

_____

?_____

_____

?_____

_____

?_____

_____

?_____

_____

?_____

_____

?_____

_____

?_____

_____

?_____

_____

?_____

_____

?_____

_____

?_____

_____

?_____

_____

CHAPTER TEN

Together

This space is for you to paste in a photograph of you and your children. Choose one together—one that always makes you laugh.

CLOSING NOTE

Parents rarely see the direct product of parenting. We preach manners, thoughtfulness, honor, charity, duty, sportsmanship and kindness, but we are seldom there when our sons and daughters face complex or challenging situations.

The most we can usually hope for is the pizza shop owner telling us that our son returned the extra dollar he had been mistakenly given in change, or the eighth-grade teacher explaining that our daughter has volunteered to act as a "big sister" to a disabled girl in kindergarten.

At these moments, we give silent thanks that somewhere during the chaos of trying to diaper two kids while making sure the other three were doing their homework, some values slipped in somewhere.

I am luckier than most. Just as I was finishing the manuscript for this book, my son Trevor—the one who looked up at me and asked, "Daddy, can I still kiss you?"—brought me the essay he had just completed for one of his college applications.

"Here," he said. "This is for you."

I have often told people that I would not wish cancer on my worst enemy, but I would not give mine back. I know that statement confuses people. Who would not wish to erase the experience of cancer? What follows explains why better than anything I could ever write.

Asked to write an essay evaluating "a significant experience and its impact on you," my son wrote the following:

Dear Department of Admissions:

I know this essay is longer than the 300 words you requested, but this is the first time I have ever written about this, and I didn't know how to make it any shorter.

COLLEGE ESSAY
A PROFOUND EFFECT

When I was in sixth grade, I was struck with the worst news of my life.

One day, my parents told my brother and me that we were going on a vacation to a hotel in Newport Beach. That seemed a little strange, since it was the middle of the school week, and even though we went to Newport Beach all the time, we never stayed in a hotel there. It was only a couple of miles from our home.

But because my father is a television and movie producer and is gone a lot, sometimes we would do things on the spur of the moment when he could take a few days off. So I just figured this was one of those times.

The day before we were going to leave, my brother and I were playing video games when my dad came up the stairs, closed the door to the family room and told us he needed to talk to us about something important. We turned off the game and began to listen, not having any idea what we were about to hear.

My dad then said straight out, "I have cancer."

I can't really explain how I felt, but after a little while, I realized that my dad was still talking but I couldn't really understand what he was saying. It was like the time in Little League when I was hit by a pitch in the cheek. As I lay on the ground, I could see my teammates and my coach looking down at me and talking, but all I could hear was my heart in my ears beating really loud.

It didn't make any sense that my dad could be sick. He seemed to be the healthiest person I knew. For as long as I can remember, he has been a health nut. He runs five miles a day, eats right and does whatever he can to stay healthy. He doesn't even get colds. How could he have cancer?

Then I heard my dad say that there was

a possibility he could die. This scared me more than anything, because I had never dealt with death before. The first thing that jumped into my mind was that my dad earned all of the money in our family and that if he did die, then we might become homeless. I know that sounds kind of self-ish, but my brain was racing all over the place.

The next day we went on our "vacation" to a hotel that was near the hospital. It was very elegant, and there were people to help us with everything, but it was all a blur to me. To this day, I don't remember what our room looked like.

My dad went in for surgery the next morning, and before he left, he hugged my brother and me and told us to go swim-ming and to just try to have a little fun. Although I could not think of having any fun because I was so worried about him.

After his surgery was over, my mom took us to visit him. I was not ready for what I saw. My dad was in the worst situation I had ever seen him in. When we walked into the room, he was asleep, and he looked very pale and really sick, not anything like the people on *ER*. He also looked a lot smaller than I remembered, and there were all kinds of needles stuck in him. Then he woke up and turned his head to look at us, revealing a large tube stitched into his neck that was being used to pump painkillers into him.

Up until this point, I had tried to be really tough. I had not cried one tear, but when I saw him, I lost it. Here I was looking at someone I thought was untouchable, my hero, totally incapacitated. My mom had to take me out of the room for a while. There was a nurse at a desk outside my dad's room, and she came over to me and explained that all of the needles in my dad were normal. She also said that the doctor thought he had gotten all of the cancer.

A week later, we brought my dad home, and that night I hit a monster home run in my Little League game. I knew it was gone when it came off the bat. I gave the ball to my dad.

And then, just when things were getting back to normal and my dad started to look like himself again, the cancer came back. My mom told us that this time even the doctors were very worried.

I don't think I realized it at the time, but I became a different person. I had always been kind of a difficult kid. I didn't do really bad stuff, but I talked a lot in class, and because I was a good athlete, sometimes I was hard on those who couldn't do the things I could. But after this, I became very quiet and kind of a loner because, besides my brother, there wasn't anyone I knew who could possibly understand what I was going through. I mean none of my friends' dads were fighting for their lives, and I didn't know how to even start to explain it to anyone.

My dad survived the cancer, but he's not

the same person he was. He still laughs like he used to and grounds me when I do something wrong, but he's not as strong as he used to be, and I kid him because sometimes he falls asleep in the middle of a movie. I always loved him, but now I see him as a man, not just my dad, and he and I are closer than we ever were.

I am not the same either. I realize now that there are more important things in life than whether or not someone can hit a home run or throw a pass for a touchdown. I have learned to take people as they are, and that life is very fragile.

Cancer is a terrible disease, but it can do good things, too.

Thank you for considering me.

Trevor Russell

RESOURCES

The following Web sites contain additional information that parents with cancer and their children might find helpful.

- *Breast Cancer: Common Reactions of Children and How to Help,* Jane Brazy, M.D., and Mary Ircink, R.N. *www.medsch.wisc.edu/ childrenshosp/childrens.html*

- National Cancer Institute. *www.nci.nih.gov*

- American Cancer Society. *www.cancer.org*

- Memorial Sloan-Kettering Cancer Center. *www.mskcc.org*

- Kidscope. *www.kidscope.org*

- Kids Konnected. *www.kidskonnected.org*

ABOUT THE AUTHOR

Neil Russell is president and CEO of Neil Russell Productions (NRP) and Site 85 Productions, television and motion picture production companies that create and acquire intellectual property rights. Russell is a member of the Writer's Guild of America and The Academy of Television Arts and Sciences and is currently working on a television series with MGM Television and motion pictures with Jerry Bruckheimer Films/Disney-Touchstone Pictures and Landscape Entertainment.

In Loving Memory of G.T.W.R.